INTERSTITIAL CYSTITIS DIET COOKBOOK

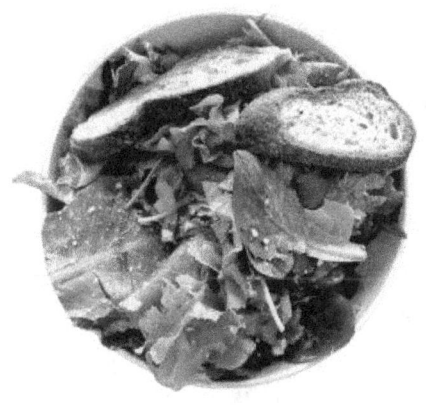

DR. JESSICA SMITH

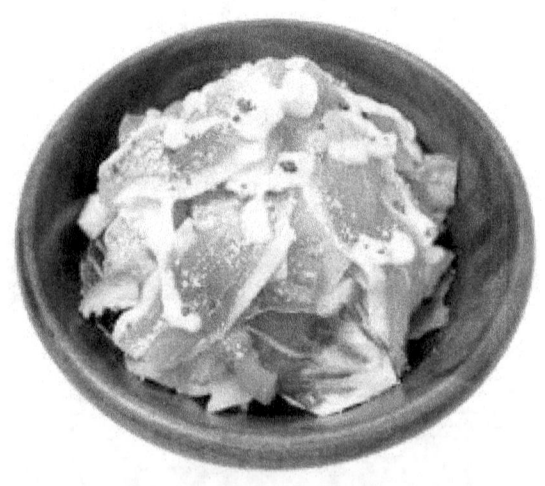

TABLE OF CONTENTS

CHAPTER ONE

How to Use this Cookbook

Understand the Condition: Before diving into the cookbook, take some time to understand interstitial cystitis (IC) and how certain foods can affect it. IC is a chronic bladder condition characterized by pain, pressure, or discomfort in the bladder and pelvic region.

Consult with a Healthcare Professional: Talk to your healthcare provider or a registered dietitian specializing in IC about dietary recommendations and restrictions that may help manage your symptoms. They can provide personalized advice tailored to your specific needs.

Review the Recipes: Take some time to browse through the recipes in the cookbook. Pay attention to the ingredients used and look for recipes that appeal to your taste preferences and dietary restrictions.

Plan Your Meals: Use the cookbook to plan your meals for the week ahead. Choose recipes that incorporate bladder-friendly ingredients and avoid known triggers such as citrus fruits, tomatoes, and artificial sweeteners.

Shop for Ingredients: Make a shopping list based on the recipes you've chosen. Be sure to include all the necessary ingredients, as well as any pantry staples you may need.

Prepare Meals Mindfully: When cooking, follow the recipes carefully and pay attention to portion sizes and cooking methods. Opt for gentle cooking techniques such as steaming, baking, or grilling, which may be easier on the bladder.

Enjoy Your Meals: Sit down and savor your meals mindfully. Pay attention to how your body responds to different foods and take note of any triggers that may exacerbate your symptoms.

Monitor Your Symptoms: Keep track of your symptoms and how they correlate with the foods you eat. If you notice any patterns or triggers, make adjustments to your diet accordingly and consult with your healthcare provider for further guidance.

Understanding Interstitial Cystitis Diet

Understanding the interstitial cystitis (IC) diet is crucial for individuals managing this chronic bladder condition. Interstitial cystitis, also known as painful bladder syndrome, is characterized by bladder pain, urinary urgency, frequency, and sometimes pelvic pain.

While the exact cause of IC is not fully understood, dietary factors play a significant role in managing symptoms for many individuals.

The IC diet aims to minimize irritation to the bladder lining by avoiding foods and beverages that may exacerbate symptoms.

Common triggers include acidic foods (such as citrus fruits and tomatoes), caffeine, spicy foods, artificial sweeteners, alcohol, and carbonated beverages. Additionally, some individuals with IC may be sensitive to certain preservatives, additives, or high-oxalate foods.

A typical IC diet focuses on consuming foods that are considered bladder-friendly, such as bland grains (like rice and oats), lean proteins (such as chicken and fish), non-citrus fruits (like pears and bananas), and vegetables (excluding those high in acids).

It also encourages adequate hydration with water and herbal teas.

However, it's important to note that not all triggers are universal, and individual tolerance varies. Some individuals may find relief by following a strict IC diet, while others may need to experiment with their food choices to identify personal triggers.

Consulting with a healthcare provider or a registered dietitian experienced in managing IC can provide personalized guidance and support in navigating the IC diet effectively.

Benefits of Interstitial Cystitis Diet

The interstitial cystitis (IC) diet offers several benefits for individuals managing this chronic bladder condition.

By following a carefully planned diet tailored to their specific needs, individuals with IC can experience significant improvements in their symptoms and overall quality of life.

One of the primary benefits of the IC diet is symptom management. By avoiding foods and beverages that may irritate the bladder lining, individuals can reduce the frequency and severity of urinary urgency, frequency, and pelvic pain associated with IC. This can lead to decreased discomfort and improved daily functioning.

Additionally, the IC diet promotes better bladder health. By consuming bladder-friendly foods and staying hydrated with water and herbal teas, individuals can support the health of their bladder lining and reduce inflammation, which may contribute to long-term symptom management and prevention of flare-ups.

Furthermore, the IC diet can help individuals regain a sense of control over their condition.

By understanding how different foods affect their symptoms and making informed dietary choices, individuals with IC can actively participate in managing their condition and feel empowered in their journey toward better health.

It's important for individuals to work closely with healthcare providers or registered dietitians to ensure that their dietary choices align with their specific needs and preferences.

Guidelines for Interstitial Cystitis Diet

Guidelines for an interstitial cystitis (IC) diet are essential for individuals seeking relief from the symptoms of this chronic bladder condition. While there is no one-size-fits-all approach, there are general principles and guidelines that can help manage symptoms and improve overall bladder health.

Firstly, individuals with IC are often advised to avoid certain foods and beverages that are known to irritate the bladder.

Common triggers include acidic foods like citrus fruits, tomatoes, and their derivatives, as well as caffeine, spicy foods, alcohol, artificial sweeteners, and carbonated beverages.

Instead, focus on incorporating bladder-friendly foods into your diet.

These include bland grains such as rice and oats, lean proteins like chicken and fish, non-citrus fruits such as pears and bananas, and vegetables excluding those high in acids.

It's also important to stay hydrated by drinking plenty of water and herbal teas, which can help flush out the bladder and reduce irritation. Meal planning plays a crucial role in adhering to the IC diet. Plan your meals around bladder-friendly ingredients and avoid known triggers. Experiment with different recipes and cooking methods to find what works best for you.

Keep a food diary to track your symptoms and identify potential triggers.

This can help you make informed decisions about your diet and lifestyle.

Finally, consult with a healthcare provider or a registered dietitian specializing in IC to develop a personalized diet plan that meets your individual needs and preferences.

Causes of Interstitial Cystitis

Interstitial cystitis (IC), also known as painful bladder syndrome, is a chronic condition characterized by bladder pain, urinary urgency, frequency, and sometimes pelvic pain.

While the exact cause of IC remains unclear, several factors are believed to contribute to its development:

Bladder Lining Defects: One theory suggests that defects in the protective lining of the bladder may play a role in the development of IC. Damage to the bladder's mucous layer allows irritants in urine to penetrate the bladder wall, leading to inflammation and pain.

Pelvic Floor Dysfunction: Dysfunction of the pelvic floor muscles, which support the bladder and other pelvic organs, may contribute to IC symptoms. Tight or tense pelvic floor muscles can cause pain and discomfort in the pelvic region.

Immune System Abnormalities: Dysfunction of the immune system may also be implicated in IC. Inflammatory processes within the bladder may be triggered by an abnormal immune response, leading to chronic inflammation and pain.

Neurogenic Inflammation: Abnormalities in the nerves that control bladder function may contribute to IC symptoms. Neurogenic inflammation, in which nerve signals trigger inflammation in the bladder, can lead to pain, urgency, and frequency.

Genetic Predisposition: There may be a genetic component to IC, as it tends to run in families. Certain genetic factors may increase susceptibility to developing the condition or predispose individuals to bladder inflammation and pain.

Other Factors: Other factors such as urinary tract infections, allergies, hormonal imbalances, and autoimmune conditions may also contribute to the development of IC.

While the exact cause of IC remains uncertain, it is likely a complex interplay of multiple factors.

Understanding these potential causes can help guide treatment and management strategies for individuals affected by this challenging condition.

Types of Interstitial Cystitis

Interstitial cystitis (IC) is a complex condition with various subtypes and manifestations, each presenting its own set of symptoms and challenges.

While the classification of IC subtypes is not universally agreed upon, several patterns and variations have been observed in clinical practice:

Classic IC: Also known as Hunner's ulcers or ulcerative IC, this subtype is characterized by visible lesions or ulcers on the bladder wall, often accompanied by intense bladder pain and urinary symptoms.

Non-ulcerative IC: This subtype does not exhibit visible ulcers or lesions on the bladder wall but shares many of the symptoms associated with classic IC, including urinary urgency, frequency, and pelvic pain.

Bladder Pain Syndrome (BPS): Some healthcare providers use the term BPS interchangeably with IC, referring to a broader spectrum of bladder pain disorders characterized by pelvic pain, urinary urgency, and frequency. BPS encompasses both ulcerative and non-ulcerative forms of IC.

Overlapping Conditions: Many individuals with IC also experience comorbid conditions such as irritable bowel syndrome (IBS), fibromyalgia, endometriosis, and chronic pelvic pain syndrome (CPPS). These overlapping conditions can complicate diagnosis and treatment.

Subclinical IC: In some cases, individuals may exhibit symptoms consistent with IC but do not meet the diagnostic criteria for a formal diagnosis. This subtype is often challenging to diagnose and manage due to the absence of definitive clinical markers.

Understanding the various types and subtypes of IC is essential for accurate diagnosis and personalized treatment planning.

A multidisciplinary approach involving healthcare providers from various specialties, including urology, gynecology, and pain management, may be necessary to effectively manage the diverse presentations of this complex condition.

Symptoms of Interstitial Cystitis

Interstitial cystitis (IC), also known as painful bladder syndrome, manifests through a variety of symptoms that can significantly impact a person's quality of life.

The symptoms of IC can vary in severity and duration, and they may fluctuate over time. Common symptoms include:

Bladder Pain: Pain in the bladder is a hallmark symptom of IC. This pain can range from mild discomfort to severe, debilitating pain and may be described as a constant ache, pressure, or burning sensation in the pelvic region.

Urinary Urgency: Individuals with IC often experience a strong and sudden urge to urinate, even when the bladder is not full. This urgency can be distressing and may lead to frequent trips to the bathroom.

Frequency: Increased urinary frequency is another common symptom of IC. Individuals may need to urinate more frequently than usual, sometimes as often as every 10-15 minutes, which can disrupt daily activities and sleep patterns.

Nocturia: Many people with IC experience nocturia, which is the need to urinate frequently during the night. This symptom can disrupt sleep and contribute to fatigue and daytime drowsiness.

Painful Intercourse: IC can cause pain or discomfort during sexual intercourse, known as dyspareunia, due to the sensitivity of the pelvic region.

Pelvic Pain: In addition, to bladder pain, individuals with IC may experience generalized pelvic pain or discomfort that radiates to the lower abdomen, back, or groin.

Other Symptoms: Some individuals with IC may also experience blood in the urine (hematuria), discomfort or pain in the urethra, and feelings of pressure in the bladder or pelvic area.

The symptoms of IC can vary from person to person and may overlap with other bladder or pelvic conditions, making diagnosis challenging. It's essential for individuals experiencing persistent urinary symptoms or pelvic pain to seek evaluation and guidance from a healthcare provider for proper diagnosis and management.

Risk Factor of Interstitial Cystitis

Interstitial cystitis (IC) is a complex condition with multifactorial origins, and while the exact cause remains elusive, several risk factors have been identified that may increase the likelihood of developing IC.

Understanding these risk factors can help individuals and healthcare providers better recognize and manage the condition. Some of the key risk factors associated with IC include:

Gender: Women are significantly more likely to develop IC than men. It's estimated that women are diagnosed with IC at a rate of 3 to 9 times higher than men. This gender disparity suggests hormonal, anatomical, or physiological differences may play a role in the development of IC.

Age: While IC can affect individuals of any age, it is most commonly diagnosed in adults, particularly those in their 30s and 40s. However, IC can also occur in children and older adults.

Genetics: There appears to be a genetic component to IC, as the condition tends to run in families. Individuals with a family history of IC or related conditions such as irritable bowel syndrome (IBS) may have an increased risk of developing the condition themselves.

Urinary Tract Infections (UTIs): Recurrent or chronic UTIs have been linked to an increased risk of IC. Chronic bladder inflammation and irritation from repeated infections may contribute to the development of IC in susceptible individuals.

Pelvic Trauma or Surgery: Previous pelvic surgeries or trauma, such as childbirth, pelvic surgery, or pelvic radiation therapy, may increase the risk of developing IC by causing damage to the bladder or pelvic structures.

Psychological Factors: Emotional stress, anxiety, depression, and other psychological factors may exacerbate IC symptoms in some individuals. While these factors may not directly cause IC, they can contribute to symptom severity and overall quality of life.

CHAPTER TWO

Interstitial Cystitis Breakfast Diet Recipes

1: Banana Oat Pancakes

Ingredients:

- 1 ripe banana
- 1/2 cup rolled oats
- 1 egg
- 1/4 teaspoon vanilla extract
- 1/4 teaspoon ground cinnamon
- Optional toppings: sliced banana, berries, pure maple syrup (avoid if sensitive to sugars)

Instructions:

- In a blender or food processor, combine the ripe banana, rolled oats, egg, vanilla extract, and ground cinnamon. Blend until smooth.
- Heat a non-stick skillet or griddle over medium heat. Lightly grease with cooking spray or a small amount of oil.

- Pour small circles of the pancake batter onto the skillet, using about 1/4 cup of batter for each pancake.

- Cook for 2-3 minutes, or until bubbles form on the surface of the pancakes and the edges begin to set.

- Flip the pancakes and cook for an additional 1-2 minutes, or until golden brown and cooked through.

- Serve the pancakes warm, topped with sliced banana, berries, or a drizzle of pure maple syrup if desired.

Health Benefits:

- Bananas are rich in potassium and fiber, which can support digestive health and provide sustained energy.

- Oats are a good source of soluble fiber, which can help regulate blood sugar levels and promote feelings of fullness.

Preparation Time: Approximately 15 minutes

2: Scrambled Tofu with Vegetables

Ingredients:

- 1/2 block of firm tofu, drained and crumbled

- 1/4 cup diced bell peppers (any color)
- 1/4 cup diced zucchini
- 1/4 cup diced tomatoes (if tolerated)
- 1 tablespoon olive oil
- 1/4 teaspoon turmeric powder
- Salt and pepper to taste

Instructions:

- Heat olive oil in a skillet over medium heat. Add diced bell peppers and zucchini, and sauté for 2-3 minutes until slightly softened.
- Add crumbled tofu to the skillet, along with turmeric powder, salt, and pepper. Cook for another 2-3 minutes, stirring occasionally.
- If tolerated, add diced tomatoes to the skillet and cook for an additional 1-2 minutes until heated through.
- Remove from heat and serve the scrambled tofu with vegetables warm.

Health Benefits: Tofu is a plant-based source of protein that is low in fat and contains essential amino acids.

- Bell peppers and zucchini are rich in vitamins, minerals, and antioxidants, which can support overall health and immune function.

Preparation Time: Approximately 10 minutes

3: Blueberry Almond Smoothie Bowl

Ingredients:

- 1 ripe banana
- 1/2 cup frozen blueberries
- 1/4 cup unsweetened almond milk (or any non-dairy milk)
- 1 tablespoon almond butter
- 1 tablespoon ground flaxseed (optional)
- Toppings: sliced almonds, fresh blueberries, shredded coconut (avoid if sensitive to coconut)

Instructions:

- In a blender, combine the ripe banana, frozen blueberries, almond milk, almond butter, and ground flaxseed (if using). Blend until smooth and creamy.
- Pour the smoothie into a bowl.

- Top with sliced almonds, fresh blueberries, and shredded coconut if desired.
- Serve immediately and enjoy with a spoon!

Health Benefits:

- Blueberries are rich in antioxidants and anti-inflammatory compounds, which can help reduce inflammation and support urinary tract health.
- Almonds and almond butter provide healthy fats, protein, and fiber, which can help stabilize blood sugar levels and promote satiety.

Preparation Time: Approximately 5 minutes

4: Quinoa Breakfast Porridge

Ingredients:

- 1/2 cup cooked quinoa
- 1/2 cup unsweetened almond milk (or any non-dairy milk)
- 1/4 teaspoon ground cinnamon
- 1 tablespoon pure maple syrup (optional, avoid if sensitive to sugars)
- 1/4 cup sliced strawberries

- 1 tablespoon chopped walnuts

Instructions:

- In a small saucepan, combine the cooked quinoa, almond milk, ground cinnamon, and pure maple syrup (if using). Heat over medium heat until warm, stirring occasionally.
- Once heated through, transfer the quinoa porridge to a bowl.
- Top with sliced strawberries and chopped walnuts.
- Serve warm and enjoy as a comforting breakfast option.

Health Benefits:

- Quinoa is a gluten-free whole grain that is rich in protein, fiber, and essential nutrients, making it a nutritious breakfast choice.
- Strawberries are low in sugar and calories but high in vitamin C and antioxidants, which can support immune health and reduce inflammation.

Preparation Time: Approximately 10 minutes

5: Avocado Toast with Poached Egg

Ingredients:

- 1 slice of whole grain bread (or gluten-free bread if needed)
- 1/2 ripe avocado, mashed
- 1 large egg
- Salt and pepper to taste
- Optional toppings: sliced cherry tomatoes, chopped chives, or a sprinkle of sesame seeds

Instructions:

- Toast the slice of whole grain bread until golden brown.
- Spread the mashed avocado evenly onto the toasted bread.
- Fill a small saucepan with water and bring it to a gentle simmer over medium heat.
- Crack the egg into a small bowl. Using a spoon, create a gentle whirlpool in the simmering water and carefully slide the egg into the center of the whirlpool.

- Poach the egg for 3-4 minutes, or until the whites are set but the yolk is still runny.
- Using a slotted spoon, carefully remove the poached egg from the water and place it on top of the avocado toast.
- Season with salt and pepper to taste, and garnish with optional toppings if desired.
- Serve immediately and enjoy!

Health Benefits:

- Avocado is a nutritious source of healthy fats, fiber, and vitamins, including vitamin E and potassium, which can support heart health and reduce inflammation.
- Eggs are rich in high-quality protein and essential nutrients such as vitamin B12 and selenium, which are important for overall health and immune function.

Preparation Time: Approximately 10 minutes

6: Greek Yogurt Parfait with Honey and Almonds

Ingredients:

- 1/2 cup plain Greek yogurt (or lactose-free yogurt if sensitive to dairy)
- 1 tablespoon honey (optional, avoid if sensitive to sugars)
- 2 tablespoons sliced almonds
- 1/4 cup fresh berries (such as strawberries, blueberries, or raspberries)

Instructions:

- In a small bowl or glass, layer the plain Greek yogurt, honey (if using), sliced almonds, and fresh berries.
- Repeat the layers until all ingredients are used, ending with a sprinkle of sliced almonds and berries on top.
- Serve immediately and enjoy!

Health Benefits: Greek yogurt is a rich source of protein and probiotics, which can support digestive health and immune function.

- Berries are low in sugar and calories but high in antioxidants, vitamins, and fiber, which can help reduce inflammation and support urinary tract health.

Preparation Time: Approximately 5 minutes

7: Chia Seed Pudding with Mixed Berries

Ingredients:

- 2 tablespoons chia seeds
- 1/2 cup unsweetened almond milk (or any non-dairy milk)
- 1/4 teaspoon vanilla extract
- 1 teaspoon pure maple syrup (optional, avoid if sensitive to sugars)
- 1/4 cup mixed berries (such as strawberries, blueberries, raspberries)
- Optional toppings: sliced almonds, shredded coconut (avoid if sensitive to coconut)

Instructions:

- In a small bowl or jar, combine the chia seeds, unsweetened almond milk, vanilla extract, and pure maple syrup (if using). Stir well to combine.

- Cover the bowl or jar and refrigerate for at least 2 hours, or overnight, to allow the chia seeds to absorb the liquid and form a pudding-like consistency.
- Once the chia pudding has set, remove it from the refrigerator and give it a stir.
- Top the chia seed pudding with mixed berries and any optional toppings you desire.
- Serve chilled and enjoy this nutritious breakfast option!

Health Benefits:

- Chia seeds are rich in fiber, omega-3 fatty acids, and antioxidants, which can support digestive health, heart health, and reduce inflammation.
- Mixed berries provide a variety of vitamins, minerals, and antioxidants, which can help support immune function and reduce oxidative stress.

Preparation Time: Approximately 5 minutes (plus chilling time)

8: Cottage Cheese and Pineapple Bowl

Ingredients:

- 1/2 cup low-fat cottage cheese (or lactose-free cottage cheese if sensitive to dairy)
- 1/2 cup diced pineapple (fresh or canned in natural juice)
- 1 tablespoon chopped walnuts
- Optional: a drizzle of honey (optional, avoid if sensitive to sugars)

Instructions:

- In a bowl, combine the low-fat cottage cheese and diced pineapple.
- Sprinkle the chopped walnuts over the top of the cottage cheese and pineapple mixture.
- If desired, drizzle a small amount of honey over the bowl for added sweetness.
- Serve immediately and enjoy this simple and satisfying breakfast option!

Health Benefits:

- Cottage cheese is a good source of protein and calcium, which are important for muscle health and bone health.
- Pineapple contains bromelain, an enzyme that may help reduce inflammation and promote digestion.

Preparation Time: Approximately 5 minutes

9: Turkey and Veggie Breakfast Scramble

Ingredients:

- 2 large eggs
- 2 slices of turkey breast, chopped
- 1/4 cup diced bell peppers (any color)
- 1/4 cup diced zucchini
- 1 tablespoon olive oil
- Salt and pepper to taste

Instructions:

- Heat olive oil in a skillet over medium heat. Add diced bell peppers and zucchini, and sauté for 2-3 minutes until slightly softened.

- Add chopped turkey breast to the skillet and cook for another 1-2 minutes, stirring occasionally.
- Crack the eggs into the skillet and scramble them with the vegetables and turkey until cooked through.
- Season with salt and pepper to taste.
- Once everything is cooked, transfer the scramble to a plate and serve immediately.

Health Benefits:

- Turkey breast is a lean source of protein, which can help promote satiety and support muscle health.
- Bell peppers and zucchini are rich in vitamins, minerals, and antioxidants, which can support overall health and reduce inflammation.

Preparation Time: Approximately 10 minutes

10: Baked Apple Oatmeal Cups

Ingredients:

- 1 cup rolled oats
- 1 large apple, grated
- 1/4 cup unsweetened applesauce

- 1/4 cup unsweetened almond milk (or any non-dairy milk)
- 1 tablespoon pure maple syrup (optional, avoid if sensitive to sugars)
- 1/2 teaspoon ground cinnamon
- 1/4 teaspoon vanilla extract
- Optional toppings: sliced almonds, a sprinkle of cinnamon

Instructions:

- Preheat your oven to 350°F (175°C). Grease a muffin tin or line with paper liners.
- In a mixing bowl, combine the rolled oats, grated apple, unsweetened applesauce, almond milk, pure maple syrup (if using), ground cinnamon, and vanilla extract. Stir until well combined.
- Divide the oatmeal mixture evenly among the muffin cups, filling each one almost to the top.
- Sprinkle sliced almonds and a little extra cinnamon on top of each oatmeal cup, if desired.

- Bake in the preheated oven for 20-25 minutes, or until the oatmeal cups are set and lightly golden brown on top.
- Allow the oatmeal cups to cool slightly before removing them from the muffin tin. Serve warm or at room temperature.

Health Benefits:

- Rolled oats are a good source of fiber, which can help promote digestive health and reduce cholesterol levels.
- Apples are rich in fiber and antioxidants, which can support heart health and reduce inflammation.
- Preparation Time: Approximately 30 minutes (including baking time)

Interstitial Cystitis Lunch Diet Recipes

1: Grilled Chicken Salad with Balsamic Vinaigrette

Ingredients:

- 2 cups mixed salad greens (such as spinach, arugula, or lettuce)

- 4 ounces grilled chicken breast, sliced
- 1/4 cup cherry tomatoes, halved
- 1/4 cup cucumber, sliced
- 1/4 cup bell peppers, sliced
- 1 tablespoon olive oil
- 1 tablespoon balsamic vinegar
- Salt and pepper to taste

Instructions:

- In a large salad bowl, combine the mixed salad greens, grilled chicken breast slices, cherry tomatoes, cucumber slices, and bell peppers.
- In a small bowl, whisk together the olive oil and balsamic vinegar to make the dressing.
- Drizzle the dressing over the salad and toss gently to coat.
- Season with salt and pepper to taste.
- Serve the grilled chicken salad immediately as a satisfying and nutritious lunch option.

Health Benefits:

- Grilled chicken breast is a lean source of protein, which can help promote satiety and support muscle health.

- Salad greens, cherry tomatoes, cucumber, and bell peppers are rich in vitamins, minerals, and antioxidants, which can support overall health and reduce inflammation.

Preparation Time: Approximately 15 minutes

2: Quinoa Salad with Lemon Herb Dressing

Ingredients:

- 1 cup cooked quinoa, cooled
- 1/2 cup cucumber, diced
- 1/2 cup cherry tomatoes, halved
- 1/4 cup red onion, finely chopped
- 2 tablespoons chopped fresh parsley
- 2 tablespoons chopped fresh mint
- 1 tablespoon olive oil
- 1 tablespoon freshly squeezed lemon juice
- Salt and pepper to taste

Instructions:

- In a large mixing bowl, combine the cooked quinoa, diced cucumber, cherry tomatoes, red onion, chopped parsley, and chopped mint.
- In a small bowl, whisk together the olive oil and lemon juice to make the dressing.
- Drizzle the dressing over the quinoa salad and toss gently to coat.
- Season with salt and pepper to taste.
- Serve the quinoa salad chilled or at room temperature as a refreshing and nutritious lunch option.

Health Benefits:

- Quinoa is a gluten-free whole grain that is rich in protein, fiber, and essential nutrients, making it a nutritious and satisfying base for salads.
- Cucumber, cherry tomatoes, red onion, parsley, and mint provide a variety of vitamins, minerals, and antioxidants, which can support overall health and reduce inflammation.

Preparation Time: Approximately 20 minutes (including cooking quinoa)

3: Salmon and Quinoa Salad

Ingredients:

- 4 ounces grilled or baked salmon fillet, flaked
- 1 cup cooked quinoa, cooled
- 1/4 cup cucumber, diced
- 1/4 cup red bell pepper, diced
- 1/4 cup carrots, shredded
- 2 tablespoons chopped fresh dill
- 1 tablespoon olive oil
- 1 tablespoon freshly squeezed lemon juice
- Salt and pepper to taste

Instructions:

- In a large mixing bowl, combine the flaked salmon, cooked quinoa, diced cucumber, diced red bell pepper, shredded carrots, and chopped fresh dill.
- In a small bowl, whisk together the olive oil and lemon juice to make the dressing.
- Drizzle the dressing over the salmon and quinoa salad and toss gently to coat.
- Season with salt and pepper to taste.

- Serve the salmon and quinoa salad chilled or at room temperature as a nutritious and satisfying lunch option.

Health Benefits:

- Salmon is a fatty fish rich in omega-3 fatty acids, which have anti-inflammatory properties and may help reduce inflammation associated with interstitial cystitis.
- Quinoa is a gluten-free whole grain that is rich in protein, fiber, and essential nutrients, providing sustained energy and promoting digestive health.
- Preparation Time: Approximately 20 minutes (including cooking quinoa and salmon)

4: Turkey Wrap with Avocado and Spinach

Ingredients:

- 1 whole grain or gluten-free tortilla wrap
- 2 ounces sliced turkey breast
- 1/4 avocado, sliced
- 1/4 cup baby spinach leaves

- 1 tablespoon hummus (optional, avoid if sensitive to legumes)
- Salt and pepper to taste

Instructions:

- Lay the tortilla wrap flat on a clean surface.
- Spread the hummus evenly over the tortilla wrap, if using.
- Layer the sliced turkey breast, avocado slices, and baby spinach leaves on top of the tortilla wrap.
- Season with salt and pepper to taste.
- Roll up the tortilla wrap tightly, tucking in the sides as you go.
- Slice the turkey wrap in half diagonally.
- Serve immediately as a convenient and portable lunch option.

Health Benefits:

- Turkey breast is a lean source of protein, which can help promote satiety and support muscle health.

- Avocado provides healthy fats and essential nutrients, including potassium and fiber, which can support heart health and reduce inflammation.

Preparation Time: Approximately 10 minutes

5: Veggie Stir-Fry with Brown Rice

Ingredients:

- 1 cup cooked brown rice, cooled
- 1/2 cup mixed vegetables (such as bell peppers, carrots, broccoli, snap peas)
- 2 tablespoons low-sodium soy sauce (or tamari for gluten-free option)
- 1 tablespoon olive oil
- 1 clove garlic, minced
- 1/2 teaspoon grated ginger
- Optional toppings: sliced green onions, sesame seeds

Instructions:

- Heat olive oil in a skillet or wok over medium-high heat.
- Add minced garlic and grated ginger to the skillet and sauté for 1-minute until fragrant.

- Add mixed vegetables to the skillet and stir-fry for 3-4 minutes until tender-crisp.
- Stir in cooked brown rice and low-sodium soy sauce (or tamari) until well combined.
- Cook for an additional 2-3 minutes, stirring occasionally, until heated through.
- Remove from heat and transfer the veggie stir-fry to a plate.
- Garnish with sliced green onions and sesame seeds, if desired.
- Serve immediately as a flavorful and nutritious lunch option.

Health Benefits:

- Brown rice is a whole grain rich in fiber, which can promote digestive health and help regulate blood sugar levels.
- Mixed vegetables provide a variety of vitamins, minerals, and antioxidants, which can support overall health and reduce inflammation.

Preparation Time: Approximately 20 minutes (including cooking rice and stir-frying vegetables)

6: Turkey and Veggie Lettuce Wraps

Ingredients:

- 4 large lettuce leaves (such as romaine or butter lettuce)
- 4 ounces cooked turkey breast, thinly sliced
- 1/4 cup shredded carrots
- 1/4 cup diced cucumber
- 1/4 cup diced bell peppers
- 2 tablespoons hummus (optional, avoid if sensitive to legumes)
- 1 tablespoon olive oil
- 1 tablespoon freshly squeezed lemon juice
- Salt and pepper to taste

Instructions:

- Lay the lettuce leaves flat on a clean surface.
- Spread a thin layer of hummus (if using) onto each lettuce leaf.
- Layer the thinly sliced turkey breast, shredded carrots, diced cucumber, and diced bell peppers on top of each lettuce leaf.

- In a small bowl, whisk together the olive oil and lemon juice to make a simple dressing.
- Drizzle the dressing over the turkey and veggie lettuce wraps.
- Season with salt and pepper to taste.
- Roll up the lettuce leaves tightly to form wraps.
- Serve immediately as a light and refreshing lunch option.

Health Benefits:

- Lettuce wraps provide a low-carb alternative to traditional wraps or sandwiches, making them suitable for individuals following a low-carb or gluten-free diet.
- Turkey breast is a lean source of protein, which can help promote satiety and support muscle health.

Preparation Time: Approximately 10 minutes

7: Quinoa and Black Bean Salad

Ingredients:

- 1 cup cooked quinoa, cooled
- 1/2 cup canned black beans, rinsed and drained

- 1/4 cup diced red bell pepper
- 1/4 cup diced cucumber
- 2 tablespoons chopped fresh cilantro
- 1 tablespoon olive oil
- 1 tablespoon freshly squeezed lime juice
- Salt and pepper to taste

Instructions:

- In a large mixing bowl, combine the cooked quinoa, black beans, diced red bell pepper, diced cucumber, and chopped fresh cilantro.
- In a small bowl, whisk together the olive oil and lime juice to make the dressing.
- Drizzle the dressing over the quinoa and black bean salad and toss gently to coat.
- Season with salt and pepper to taste.
- Serve the quinoa and black bean salad chilled or at room temperature as a flavorful and nutritious lunch option.

Health Benefits:

- Quinoa is a gluten-free whole grain that is rich in protein, fiber, and essential nutrients, making it a nutritious and satisfying base for salads.
- Black beans are a good source of plant-based protein and fiber, which can help promote satiety and support digestive health.

Preparation Time: Approximately 15 minutes (including cooking quinoa)

8: Tuna Salad Lettuce Wraps

Ingredients:

- 1 can (5 ounces) tuna in water, drained
- 2 tablespoons plain Greek yogurt (or mayonnaise if tolerated)
- 1 tablespoon finely chopped red onion
- 1 tablespoon chopped fresh parsley
- 1 tablespoon freshly squeezed lemon juice
- Salt and pepper to taste
- 4 large lettuce leaves (such as romaine or iceberg)
- Optional toppings: sliced avocado, diced tomatoes

Instructions:

- In a mixing bowl, combine the drained tuna, plain Greek yogurt (or mayonnaise), finely chopped red onion, chopped fresh parsley, and freshly squeezed lemon juice.
- Season with salt and pepper to taste and mix until well combined.
- Lay the lettuce leaves flat on a clean surface.
- Spoon the tuna salad mixture onto each lettuce leaf.
- Top with optional toppings such as sliced avocado and diced tomatoes, if desired.
- Roll up the lettuce leaves tightly to form wraps.
- Serve immediately as a protein-packed and refreshing lunch option.

Health Benefits:

- Tuna is a lean source of protein and omega-3 fatty acids, which have anti-inflammatory properties and may help reduce inflammation associated with interstitial cystitis.

- Greek yogurt is a good source of protein and probiotics, which can support digestive health and immune function.

Preparation Time: Approximately 10 minutes

9: Egg Salad Lettuce Wraps

Ingredients:

- 4 large lettuce leaves (such as romaine or butter lettuce)
- 4 hard-boiled eggs, peeled and chopped
- 2 tablespoons plain Greek yogurt
- 1 tablespoon Dijon mustard
- 1 tablespoon finely chopped chives
- Salt and pepper to taste
- Optional toppings: sliced cucumber, alfalfa sprouts

Instructions:

- Lay the lettuce leaves flat on a clean surface.
- In a mixing bowl, combine the chopped hard-boiled eggs, plain Greek yogurt, Dijon mustard, finely chopped chives, salt, and pepper.

- Mix well until all ingredients are thoroughly combined.
- Spoon the egg salad mixture onto each lettuce leaf.
- Top with optional toppings such as sliced cucumber and alfalfa sprouts, if desired.
- Roll up the lettuce leaves tightly to form wraps.
- Serve immediately as a protein-rich and satisfying lunch option.

Health Benefits:

- Eggs are a good source of high-quality protein and essential nutrients such as vitamin B12 and choline, which are important for brain health and metabolism.
- Greek yogurt provides additional protein and probiotics, which can support digestive health and immune function.

Preparation Time: Approximately 15 minutes (including boiling eggs)

10: Turkey and Avocado Wrap

Ingredients:

- 1 whole grain or gluten-free tortilla wrap

- 2 ounces sliced turkey breast
- 1/4 avocado, sliced
- 1/4 cup baby spinach leaves
- 1 tablespoon hummus (optional, avoid if sensitive to legumes)
- Salt and pepper to taste

Instructions:

- Lay the tortilla wrap flat on a clean surface.
- Spread a thin layer of hummus (if using) onto the tortilla wrap.
- Layer the sliced turkey breast, avocado slices, and baby spinach leaves on top of the tortilla wrap.
- Season with salt and pepper to taste.
- Roll up the tortilla wrap tightly, tucking in the sides as you go.
- Slice the turkey wrap in half diagonally.
- Serve immediately as a convenient and satisfying lunch option.

Health Benefits:

- Turkey breast is a lean source of protein, which can help promote satiety and support muscle health.

- Avocado provides healthy fats and essential nutrients, including potassium and fiber, which can support heart health and reduce inflammation.

Preparation Time: Approximately 10 minutes

Interstitial Cystitis Dinner Diet Recipes

1: Baked Salmon with Lemon Herb Quinoa

Ingredients:

- 2 salmon fillets (4-6 ounces each)
- 1 cup quinoa
- 2 cups low-sodium chicken or vegetable broth
- 1 tablespoon olive oil
- 1 tablespoon freshly squeezed lemon juice
- 1 teaspoon dried dill
- Salt and pepper to taste
- Optional: Lemon slices and fresh herbs for garnish

Instructions:

- Preheat the oven to 375°F (190°C).
- Rinse the quinoa under cold water in a fine mesh sieve.

- In a saucepan, bring the chicken or vegetable broth to a boil. Add the rinsed quinoa, reduce heat to low, cover, and simmer for 15-20 minutes, or until the quinoa is tender and the liquid is absorbed.
- While the quinoa is cooking, place the salmon fillets on a baking sheet lined with parchment paper or aluminum foil. Drizzle with olive oil and freshly squeezed lemon juice.
- Sprinkle dried dill, salt, and pepper over the salmon fillets.
- Bake the salmon in the preheated oven for 12-15 minutes, or until the salmon is cooked through and flakes easily with a fork.
- Once the quinoa is cooked, fluff it with a fork and season with salt and pepper to taste.
- Serve the baked salmon alongside the lemon herb quinoa. Garnish with lemon slices and fresh herbs if desired.

Health Benefits: Salmon is rich in omega-3 fatty acids, which have anti-inflammatory properties and may help reduce inflammation associated with interstitial cystitis.

- Quinoa is a gluten-free whole grain that is high in protein, fiber, and essential nutrients, providing sustained energy and supporting digestive health.

Preparation Time: Approximately 30 minutes

2: Turkey and Vegetable Stir-Fry

Ingredients:

- 1 tablespoon olive oil
- 1 pound ground turkey
- 2 cloves garlic, minced
- 1 teaspoon grated ginger
- 2 cups mixed vegetables (such as bell peppers, broccoli, carrots, snap peas)
- 2 tablespoons low-sodium soy sauce (or tamari for gluten-free option)
- 1 tablespoon honey (optional, avoid if sensitive to sugars)
- Cooked brown rice or quinoa for serving

Instructions:

- Heat olive oil in a large skillet or wok over medium-high heat.

- Add ground turkey to the skillet and cook until browned, breaking it up with a spatula as it cooks.
- Add minced garlic and grated ginger to the skillet and cook for 1 minute until fragrant.
- Add mixed vegetables to the skillet and stir-fry for 3-4 minutes until tender-crisp.
- In a small bowl, whisk together low-sodium soy sauce and honey (if using).
- Pour the sauce over the turkey and vegetables in the skillet and stir to combine.
- Continue to cook for an additional 2-3 minutes until the sauce thickens slightly and coats the turkey and vegetables.
- Serve the turkey and vegetable stir-fry hot over cooked brown rice or quinoa.

Health Benefits:

- Ground turkey is a lean source of protein, which can help promote satiety and support muscle health.
- Mixed vegetables provide a variety of vitamins, minerals, and antioxidants, which can support overall health and reduce inflammation.

Preparation Time: Approximately 25 minutes

3: Grilled Chicken with Roasted Vegetables

Ingredients:

- 2 boneless, skinless chicken breasts
- 2 cups mixed vegetables (such as zucchini, bell peppers, cherry tomatoes)
- 2 tablespoons olive oil
- 1 teaspoon dried Italian seasoning
- Salt and pepper to taste
- Optional: Balsamic glaze for serving

Instructions:

- Preheat the grill to medium-high heat.
- Season the chicken breasts with dried Italian seasoning, salt, and pepper.
- Drizzle the mixed vegetables with olive oil and season with salt and pepper.
- Place the chicken breasts and mixed vegetables on the grill.
- Grill the chicken for 6-8 minutes per side, or until cooked through and no longer pink in the center.

- Grill the mixed vegetables for 8-10 minutes, or until tender and lightly charred, flipping occasionally.
- Once the chicken is cooked through and the vegetables are tender, remove them from the grill.
- Serve the grilled chicken alongside the roasted vegetables.
- Drizzle with balsamic glaze, if desired, for added flavor.

Health Benefits:

- Chicken breast is a lean source of protein, which can help promote satiety and support muscle health.
- Mixed vegetables are rich in vitamins, minerals, and antioxidants, which can support overall health and reduce inflammation.

Preparation Time: Approximately 20 minutes

4: Shrimp and Vegetable Stir-Fry

Ingredients:

- 1 tablespoon olive oil
- 1 pound shrimp, peeled and deveined

- 2 cups mixed vegetables (such as broccoli, bell peppers, snap peas, carrots)
- 2 cloves garlic, minced
- 1 teaspoon grated ginger
- 2 tablespoons low-sodium soy sauce (or tamari for gluten-free option)
- 1 tablespoon rice vinegar
- 1 teaspoon sesame oil
- Cooked brown rice or quinoa for serving

Instructions:

- Heat olive oil in a large skillet or wok over medium-high heat.
- Add shrimp to the skillet and cook for 2-3 minutes per side until pink and opaque. Remove shrimp from the skillet and set aside.
- In the same skillet, add mixed vegetables, minced garlic, and grated ginger. Stir-fry for 3-4 minutes until vegetables are tender-crisp.
- Return the cooked shrimp to the skillet.

- In a small bowl, whisk together low-sodium soy sauce, rice vinegar, and sesame oil. Pour the sauce over the shrimp and vegetables in the skillet.
- Stir to coat everything evenly in the sauce and cook for an additional 1-2 minutes until heated through.
- Serve the shrimp and vegetable stir-fry hot over cooked brown rice or quinoa.

Health Benefits:

- Shrimp is a low-calorie source of protein and omega-3 fatty acids, which can help reduce inflammation and support heart health.
- Mixed vegetables provide fiber, vitamins, and minerals, which can support digestive health and reduce inflammation.

Preparation Time: Approximately 25 minutes

5: Turkey and Sweet Potato Hash

Ingredients:

- 1 tablespoon olive oil
- 1 pound ground turkey
- 2 medium sweet potatoes, peeled and diced

- 1 bell pepper, diced
- 1 onion, diced
- 2 cloves garlic, minced
- 1 teaspoon ground cumin
- 1 teaspoon paprika
- Salt and pepper to taste
- Fresh parsley or cilantro for garnish (optional)

Instructions:

- Heat olive oil in a large skillet over medium heat.
- Add ground turkey to the skillet and cook until browned, breaking it up with a spatula as it cooks.
- Add diced sweet potatoes, bell pepper, and onion to the skillet. Cook for 8-10 minutes, or until the sweet potatoes are tender.
- Add minced garlic, ground cumin, paprika, salt, and pepper to the skillet. Stir well to combine.
- Continue to cook for another 2-3 minutes, allowing the flavors to meld together.
- Taste and adjust seasoning if needed.
- Serve the turkey and sweet potato hash hot, garnished with fresh parsley or cilantro if desired.

Health Benefits:

- Sweet potatoes are rich in fiber, vitamins, and antioxidants, which can support digestive health and reduce inflammation.
- Turkey is a lean source of protein, which can help promote satiety and support muscle health.

Preparation Time: Approximately 30 minutes

6: Baked Cod with Lemon Herb Quinoa

Ingredients:

- 2 cod fillets (4-6 ounces each)
- 1 cup quinoa
- 2 cups low-sodium chicken or vegetable broth
- 2 tablespoons olive oil
- 1 tablespoon freshly squeezed lemon juice
- 1 teaspoon dried thyme
- Salt and pepper to taste
- Lemon wedges for serving

Instructions:

- Preheat the oven to 375°F (190°C).

- Rinse the quinoa under cold water in a fine mesh sieve.
- In a saucepan, bring the chicken or vegetable broth to a boil. Add the rinsed quinoa, reduce heat to low, cover, and simmer for 15-20 minutes, or until the quinoa is tender and the liquid is absorbed.
- While the quinoa is cooking, place the cod fillets on a baking sheet lined with parchment paper or aluminum foil. Drizzle with olive oil and freshly squeezed lemon juice.
- Sprinkle dried thyme, salt, and pepper over the cod fillets.
- Bake the cod in the preheated oven for 12-15 minutes, or until the fish is cooked through and flakes easily with a fork.
- Once the quinoa is cooked, fluff it with a fork and season with salt and pepper to taste.
- Serve the baked cod alongside the lemon herb quinoa, with lemon wedges on the side for squeezing over the fish.

Health Benefits:

- Cod is a lean source of protein and omega-3 fatty acids, which can help reduce inflammation and support heart health.
- Quinoa is a gluten-free whole grain that is high in protein, fiber, and essential nutrients, providing sustained energy and supporting digestive health.

Preparation Time: Approximately 30 minutes

7: Turkey and Vegetable Soup

Ingredients:

- 1 tablespoon olive oil
- 1 pound ground turkey
- 1 onion, diced
- 2 carrots, diced
- 2 celery stalks, diced
- 2 cloves garlic, minced
- 6 cups low-sodium chicken or vegetable broth
- 1 teaspoon dried thyme
- 1 teaspoon dried rosemary
- Salt and pepper to taste

- Fresh parsley for garnish (optional)

Instructions:

- Heat olive oil in a large pot over medium heat.
- Add ground turkey to the pot and cook until browned, breaking it up with a spatula as it cooks.
- Add diced onion, carrots, and celery to the pot. Cook for 5-7 minutes, or until vegetables are softened.
- Add minced garlic, dried thyme, and dried rosemary to the pot. Cook for 1 minute until fragrant.
- Pour in the chicken or vegetable broth and bring the soup to a simmer.
- Reduce heat to low and let the soup simmer for 20-25 minutes, allowing the flavors to meld together.
- Taste and adjust seasoning with salt and pepper if needed.
- Serve the turkey and vegetable soup hot, garnished with fresh parsley if desired.

Health Benefits:

- Turkey is a lean source of protein, which can help promote satiety and support muscle health.

- Vegetables provide fiber, vitamins, and minerals, which can support digestive health and reduce inflammation.

Preparation Time: Approximately 40 minutes

8: Baked Chicken and Vegetable Casserole

Ingredients:

- 2 boneless, skinless chicken breasts
- 2 cups mixed vegetables (such as broccoli, cauliflower, bell peppers)
- 1 tablespoon olive oil
- 1 teaspoon garlic powder
- 1 teaspoon dried Italian seasoning
- Salt and pepper to taste

Instructions:

- Preheat the oven to 375°F (190°C). Grease a baking dish with olive oil or non-stick cooking spray.
- Place the chicken breasts in the prepared baking dish.
- Arrange the mixed vegetables around the chicken breasts in the baking dish.

- Drizzle olive oil over the chicken breasts and vegetables.
- Sprinkle garlic powder, dried Italian seasoning, salt, and pepper over the chicken breasts and vegetables.
- Cover the baking dish with aluminum foil and bake in the preheated oven for 25-30 minutes, or until the chicken is cooked through and the vegetables are tender.
- Remove the foil during the last 10 minutes of baking to allow the chicken and vegetables to brown slightly.
- Serve the baked chicken and vegetable casserole hot, with your choice of side dish.

Health Benefits:

- Chicken breast is a lean source of protein, which can help promote satiety and support muscle health.
- Mixed vegetables provide fiber, vitamins, and minerals, which can support digestive health and reduce inflammation.

Preparation Time: Approximately 35 minutes

9: Turkey and Quinoa Stuffed Bell Peppers

Ingredients:

- 4 large bell peppers (any color), tops removed and seeds removed
- 1 tablespoon olive oil
- 1 onion, diced
- 2 cloves garlic, minced
- 1-pound ground turkey
- 1 cup cooked quinoa
- 1 cup diced tomatoes (canned or fresh)
- 1 teaspoon dried oregano
- 1 teaspoon dried basil
- Salt and pepper to taste
- Grated cheese for topping (optional)

Instructions:

- Preheat the oven to 375°F (190°C).
- Heat olive oil in a skillet over medium heat. Add diced onion and minced garlic, and cook until softened, about 5 minutes.

- Add ground turkey to the skillet and cook until browned, breaking it up with a spatula as it cooks.
- Stir in cooked quinoa, diced tomatoes, dried oregano, dried basil, salt, and pepper. Cook for an additional 2-3 minutes until heated through.
- Stuff each bell pepper with the turkey and quinoa mixture.
- Place stuffed bell peppers upright in a baking dish. Cover the dish with aluminum foil.
- Bake in the preheated oven for 25-30 minutes, or until the bell peppers are tender.
- If desired, sprinkle grated cheese over the stuffed bell peppers during the last 5 minutes of baking.
- Serve the turkey and quinoa stuffed bell peppers hot, garnished with fresh herbs if desired.

Health Benefits:

- Bell peppers are low in calories and rich in vitamins C and A, which can support immune function and reduce inflammation.

- Quinoa is a gluten-free whole grain that is high in protein, fiber, and essential nutrients, providing sustained energy and supporting digestive health.

Preparation Time: Approximately 45 minutes

10: Baked Cod with Roasted Vegetables

Ingredients:

- 2 cod fillets (4-6 ounces each)
- 2 cups mixed vegetables (such as cherry tomatoes, zucchini, bell peppers)
- 2 tablespoons olive oil
- 1 teaspoon dried thyme
- 1 teaspoon dried rosemary
- Salt and pepper to taste
- Lemon wedges for serving

Instructions:

- Preheat the oven to 375°F (190°C).
- Place the cod fillets on a baking sheet lined with parchment paper or aluminum foil.

- In a mixing bowl, toss the mixed vegetables with olive oil, dried thyme, dried rosemary, salt, and pepper until evenly coated.
- Spread the seasoned vegetables around the cod fillets on the baking sheet.
- Bake in the preheated oven for 15-20 minutes, or until the cod is cooked through and flakes easily with a fork, and the vegetables are tender.
- Remove from the oven and serve the baked cod with roasted vegetables hot, with lemon wedges on the side for squeezing over the fish.

Health Benefits:

- Cod is a lean source of protein and omega-3 fatty acids, which can help reduce inflammation and support heart health.
- Mixed vegetables provide fiber, vitamins, and minerals, which can support digestive health and reduce inflammation.

Preparation Time: Approximately 25 minutes

Interstitial Cystitis Snacks Recipes

1: Cucumber Hummus Bites

Ingredients:

- 1 cucumber
- 1/2 cup hummus (store-bought or homemade)
- Optional toppings: sliced cherry tomatoes, chopped fresh parsley, black olives

Instructions:

- Wash the cucumber and slice it into thick rounds, about 1/2 inch thick.
- Use a small spoon or melon baller to scoop out a small portion of the seeds from each cucumber round, creating a small well in the center.
- Fill each cucumber round with a dollop of hummus, using a spoon or piping bag.
- Top each cucumber hummus bite with optional toppings such as sliced cherry tomatoes, chopped fresh parsley, or black olives.
- Arrange the cucumber hummus bites on a serving platter and serve immediately.

Health Benefits:

- Cucumbers are low in calories and high in water content, helping to keep you hydrated and promote healthy digestion.
- Hummus is a good source of plant-based protein and fiber, which can help keep you feeling full and satisfied between meals.

Preparation Time: Approximately 10 minutes

2: Greek Yogurt Fruit Parfait

Ingredients:

- 1 cup plain Greek yogurt
- 1/2 cup mixed berries (such as strawberries, blueberries, raspberries)
- 1/4 cup granola (choose a low-sugar or homemade variety)
- 1 tablespoon honey (optional, avoid if sensitive to sugars)

Instructions:

- In a glass or bowl, layer plain Greek yogurt, mixed berries, and granola.

- Drizzle honey over the top if desired, for added sweetness.
- Repeat layering until all ingredients are used, ending with a sprinkle of granola on top.
- Serve the Greek yogurt fruit parfait immediately, or cover and refrigerate until ready to eat.

Health Benefits:

- Greek yogurt is rich in protein and probiotics, which can support digestive health and promote a healthy gut microbiome.
- Mixed berries are high in antioxidants and fiber, which can help reduce inflammation and support overall health.

Preparation Time: Approximately 5 minutes

3: Rice Cake with Avocado and Tomato

Ingredients:

- 2 rice cakes (choose a plain or low-sodium variety)
- 1/2 avocado, mashed
- 1 small tomato, sliced
- Salt and pepper to taste

- Optional toppings: fresh basil leaves, balsamic glaze

Instructions:

- Spread mashed avocado evenly onto each rice cake.
- Top the avocado-covered rice cakes with slices of tomato.
- Season with salt and pepper to taste.
- Garnish with fresh basil leaves and drizzle with balsamic glaze if desired.
- Serve the rice cakes with avocado and tomato immediately.

Health Benefits:

- Rice cakes provide a low-calorie, gluten-free base for this snack, making them suitable for individuals with interstitial cystitis.
- Avocado is rich in healthy fats and fiber, which can help promote satiety and support heart health.
- Tomatoes are a good source of vitamins C and K, as well as antioxidants like lycopene, which can help reduce inflammation and support overall health.

Preparation Time: Approximately 5 minutes

4: Cottage Cheese and Pineapple Bowl

Ingredients:

- 1/2 cup low-fat cottage cheese
- 1/2 cup fresh pineapple chunks
- Optional toppings: shredded coconut, chopped nuts (such as almonds or walnuts)

Instructions:

- In a bowl, layer low-fat cottage cheese and fresh pineapple chunks.
- Sprinkle shredded coconut and chopped nuts over the top if desired.
- Serve the cottage cheese and pineapple bowl immediately.

Health Benefits:

- Cottage cheese is a good source of protein and calcium, which can help support muscle health and bone density.
- Pineapple contains bromelain, an enzyme with anti-inflammatory properties that may help reduce inflammation associated with interstitial cystitis.

- Shredded coconut and chopped nuts provide healthy fats and additional nutrients, adding texture and flavor to the snack.

Preparation Time: Approximately 5 minutes

5: Almond Butter and Banana Rice Cakes

Ingredients:

- 2 rice cakes (choose a plain or low-sodium variety)
- 2 tablespoons almond butter (or any nut butter of your choice)
- 1 ripe banana, sliced
- Optional toppings: cinnamon, honey (optional, avoid if sensitive to sugars)

Instructions:

- Spread almond butter evenly onto each rice cake.
- Top the almond butter-covered rice cakes with slices of ripe banana.
- Sprinkle cinnamon over the top if desired.
- Drizzle with honey for added sweetness, if desired.
- Serve the almond butter and banana rice cakes immediately.

Health Benefits:

- Rice cakes provide a low-calorie, gluten-free base for this snack, making them suitable for individuals with interstitial cystitis.
- Almond butter is rich in healthy fats, protein, and fiber, which can help keep you feeling full and satisfied between meals.
- Bananas are a good source of potassium and vitamin B6, which can help support heart health and regulate blood pressure.

Preparation Time: Approximately 5 minutes

6: Veggie Sticks with Hummus

Ingredients:

- Assorted raw vegetables (such as carrots, cucumber, bell peppers, celery)
- 1/2 cup hummus (store-bought or homemade)

Instructions:

- Wash and cut assorted raw vegetables into sticks or slices.
- Arrange the vegetable sticks on a serving platter.

- Serve the vegetable sticks with hummus for dipping.

Health Benefits:

- Raw vegetables are low in calories and high in vitamins, minerals, and antioxidants, which can support overall health and reduce inflammation.
- Hummus is a good source of plant-based protein and fiber, which can help keep you feeling full and satisfied between meals.

Preparation Time: Approximately 10 minutes

7: Greek Yogurt and Berry Smoothie

Ingredients:

- 1/2 cup plain Greek yogurt
- 1/2 cup mixed berries (such as strawberries, blueberries, raspberries)
- 1/2 banana
- 1/2 cup unsweetened almond milk (or any milk of your choice)
- Optional: 1 tablespoon honey (optional, avoid if sensitive to sugars)

Instructions:

- In a blender, combine plain Greek yogurt, mixed berries, banana, and unsweetened almond milk.
- Blend until smooth and creamy.
- Taste the smoothie and add honey if desired for added sweetness.
- Pour the smoothie into a glass and serve immediately.

Health Benefits:

- Greek yogurt is rich in protein and probiotics, which can support digestive health and promote a healthy gut microbiome.
- Mixed berries are high in antioxidants and fiber, which can help reduce inflammation and support overall health.
- Banana adds natural sweetness and provides potassium, which can help regulate blood pressure and support heart health.

Preparation Time: Approximately 5 minutes

8: Cottage Cheese and Veggie Dip

Ingredients:

- 1/2 cup low-fat cottage cheese
- 1/4 cup diced cucumber
- 1/4 cup diced bell pepper
- 1 tablespoon chopped fresh dill
- Salt and pepper to taste
- Optional: Sliced raw vegetables for dipping (such as carrot sticks, celery sticks, cucumber slices)

Instructions:

- In a small bowl, combine low-fat cottage cheese, diced cucumber, diced bell pepper, and chopped fresh dill.
- Season with salt and pepper to taste.
- Stir until well combined.
- Serve the cottage cheese and veggie dip with sliced raw vegetables for dipping.

Health Benefits: Cottage cheese is a good source of protein and calcium, which can help support muscle health and bone density.

- Cucumber and bell pepper provide hydration and are low in calories, making them ideal for snacking.
- Fresh dill adds flavor and contains antioxidants, which can help reduce inflammation and support overall health.

Preparation Time: Approximately 5 minutes

9: Rice Cake with Cottage Cheese and Berries

Ingredients:

- 2 rice cakes (choose a plain or low-sodium variety)
- 1/2 cup low-fat cottage cheese
- 1/2 cup mixed berries (such as strawberries, blueberries, raspberries)
- Optional toppings: drizzle of honey (optional, avoid if sensitive to sugars), sliced almonds or walnuts

Instructions:

- Spread low-fat cottage cheese evenly onto each rice cake.
- Top the cottage cheese-covered rice cakes with mixed berries.

- Drizzle honey over the top if desired for added sweetness.
- Sprinkle sliced almonds or walnuts over the berries for added crunch.
- Serve the rice cakes with cottage cheese and berries immediately.

Health Benefits:

- Rice cakes provide a low-calorie, gluten-free base for this snack, making them suitable for individuals with interstitial cystitis.
- Cottage cheese is a good source of protein and calcium, which can help support muscle health and bone density.
- Berries are high in antioxidants and fiber, which can help reduce inflammation and support overall health.

Preparation Time: Approximately 5 minutes

10: Turkey Roll-Ups with Avocado
Ingredients:

- 4 slices low-sodium turkey breast
- 1/2 avocado, thinly sliced
- 1/4 cup baby spinach leaves

- Optional: mustard or hummus for spreading

Instructions:

- Lay out the turkey slices on a clean surface.
- Spread a thin layer of mustard or hummus (if using) onto each turkey slice.
- Place avocado slices and baby spinach leaves on top of the turkey slices.
- Roll up each turkey slice tightly to form roll-ups.
- Secure the roll-ups with toothpicks if needed.
- Serve the turkey roll-ups with avocado immediately, or refrigerate until ready to eat.

Health Benefits:

- Low-sodium turkey breast is a lean source of protein, which can help promote satiety and support muscle health.

- Avocado provides healthy fats and essential nutrients, including potassium and fiber, which can support heart health and reduce inflammation.

- Baby spinach leaves are low in calories and high in vitamins, minerals, and antioxidants, making them a nutritious addition to this snack.

Preparation Time: Approximately 10 minutes

CONCLUSION

The Interstitial Cystitis Diet Cookbook serves as an invaluable resource for individuals navigating the challenges of managing interstitial cystitis.

With its comprehensive array of bladder-friendly recipes, carefully crafted to minimize triggers and promote bladder health, this cookbook offers more than just culinary inspiration—it's a guide to reclaiming control over one's diet and well-being.

By embracing the principles outlined in this cookbook, readers can embark on a journey towards improved quality of life.

Each recipe is thoughtfully curated to prioritize ingredients that soothe rather than exacerbate symptoms, empowering individuals to make informed choices about their nutrition without sacrificing flavor or satisfaction.

Beyond its practical utility, the Interstitial Cystitis Diet Cookbook embodies a spirit of community and support. It recognizes the unique challenges faced by those living with interstitial cystitis and provides a sense of solidarity through shared experiences and collective solutions.

As readers explore the diverse range of recipes, they'll discover not only nourishment for the body but also nourishment for the soul—a renewed sense of hope, resilience, and empowerment in the face of a challenging condition.

With its wealth of culinary delights and insightful guidance, this cookbook is not just a recipe collection but a companion on the journey towards optimal health and well-being.